INSOMNIA

10 Sure Techniques to Fall Asleep & Stay Asleep For a Good Night's Rest (Cure Your Insomnia Without Drugs and Medication)

By JOSHUA ELANS

Table of Contents

Introduction

Insomnia is a condition that is characterized by difficulty falling asleep, staying asleep and feeling rested after waking up. Insomnia can also cause you to wake up in the morning early and inhibit your concentration due to prolonged tiredness.

Despite the startling ruin that insomnia can cause, a huge amount of insomniacs waits years before properly addressing their problem. Society, to a certain extent, glorifies a lack of sleep and many individuals are often met with a lack of empathy when they express how much they are suffering. It's only a lack of sleep, right?

Yet all those lost hours add up. It's hard for a well-rested person to understand the sheer apathy and despair that losing hundreds of hours of sleep can cause. Sleep is a necessary biological process, during which our mind and body are repaired. Poor sleep essentially leads to gradual decay of the mind, which becomes less efficient. Memory, willpower, concentration, emotions – everything becomes unpleasant, numb, difficult. Normal functioning is impossible.

Another reason why insomnia is so prevalent and takes so long to address is that the causes of insomnia are numerous. Poor sleep hygiene can make it difficult to achieve sleep whilst a poor lifestyle can put you on the edge and make relaxation impossible. Stress and anxiety also decimate your peace of mind, making it difficult to quell your worries and let your mind drift into oblivion. Finally, insomnia can also be a side effect of various medicines and treatments for other conditions.

Throughout our lives, it is normal to experience small bouts of insomnia, especially when we are feeling particularly stressed or anxious. Yet many people make the mistake of underestimating the extent of their own symptoms. Everyone has had a few bad nights sleep and we all understand, to a degree, just how sluggish and horrible a little tiredness can be.

Yet there is a huge difference between missing a handful of hours of sleep and missing so many that you lose count. You are not weak or whiny if you suffer from chronic insomnia, you merely need help.

Fortunately, this guide exists to provide you with 10 tried and tested ways to reliably snag some great shut eye. From improving your sleep hygiene to learning how to properly relax or even conditioning your brain to associate your bed with sleep, there are several ways in which you can make getting to sleep easier. By the time you have finished reading this guide you should be on your way to making your insomnia a thing of the past.

Chapter 1: Sleep Scheduling

Whenever people refer to their 'body clock' they are not just being metaphorical. Our bodies have evolutionary systems designed to regulate our sleeping patterns and ensure that we are awake during the day and asleep at night time.

However, our body clock needs consistency and regularity to adjust, a fact which we often ignore or fail to appreciate. Ultimately the basis of a good sleep routine is going to bed at roughly the same time every day and waking up at the same time every morning.

If you are used to an irregular sleep pattern, this will be difficult to start with and you may feel rather fatigued. Nonetheless, in the long-term a regular sleeping pattern will do wonders for helping your insomnia and you will need to push past this initial brain fog and energy deficit to reap the benefits.

In psychology and biological sciences, our sleeping patterns are dictated by our circadian rhythm (the so-called body clock mentioned earlier). The circadian rhythm is a pattern of bodily activity that cycles every 24 hours, and it includes all the various processes that make you sleep successfully, such as the release of hormones.

The important part of the circadian rhythm is the fact that it adjusts to light. In particular, natural light influences the production of the hormone *melatonin,* which dictates when we feel tired. If you fail to receive enough light on your skin, or you receive it at the wrong times, your body will produce melatonin at inconvenient times, causing you to feel tired during the day and awake during the night.

However, by knowing this fact you can take care to ensure you manage your exposure to light. Taking a few moments as you awake in the morning to bask in natural light will tell your body that you should be awake and alert during those hours. After a few days and weeks, your body will automatically adjust your circadian rhythm and melatonin release to accommodate for this information. Similarly, avoiding over-exposure to light, particularly before you go to bed is also crucial. This is why, as we will mention again later, it is best to avoid light from computers and electrical devices.

Additionally, you should consider replacing light bulbs in your house, especially in your bedroom, with light bulbs that release white light (or low blue-light light bulbs). Artificial light has a different wavelength from natural light, as it typically involves a disproportionate amount of color from the blue spectrum. This artificial light influences your melatonin release and circadian rhythm differently from natural light, adversely affecting your sleep routines.

Finally, avoid taking naps during the day, especially after 3 pm. Naps also interfere with your overall circadian rhythm, but they also ensure that you are not actually tired when you should be going to sleep. If you desperately need a nap, take a 'power nap' of no more than 30 minutes.

Chapter 2: Avoid Caffeine, Nicotine, and Alcohol

Sleep is influenced by a vast range of lifestyle choices. For example, most people are aware of the fact that caffeine is a stimulant and can prevent you from going to sleep.

Yet fewer people are aware of how caffeine can need 6-8 hours for your metabolism to fully process it and *longer if caffeine is already in your system.* The result is that for people who regularly consume too much caffeine, there is a caffeine build up in their system and they reach a critical point where their bodies are always stimulated. This leads to constantly being 'on-edge', producing a large amount stress and anxiety. Combined with inherent stimulating effects of caffeine, it is no wonder that it becomes almost impossible to get a good night's sleep.

Additionally, people are often unaware of the adverse effects of nicotine and alcohol. Nicotine is also a stimulant and it can accumulate in the body just as caffeine can, with the same dire consequences.

Alcohol is actually a depressant and doesn't prevent you from sleeping, but it does lower the quality of your sleep drastically. To be more specific, alcohol prevents REM sleep, or rapid eye movement sleep, which is considered important for long-term memory, learning and overall brain function. Alcohol also makes it much easier to wake up from a deep sleep, which is why people often find they wake up particularly early in the morning the day after they have been drinking. If you do this persistently, you'll find you reduce the number of hours you actually spend sleeping quite considerably.

On top of this, alcohol relaxes the muscles in the throat and mouth, which contributes to snoring. Above and beyond making your spouse infuriated, snoring reduces the amount of oxygen which enters your body, which once again hurts the quality of your sleep.

You don't need to live like a monk and abstain from the booze, but you do need to limit your intake, especially before bedtime. A unit of alcohol takes the average person around 1 hour for their body to process. A typical beer will usually be 1 unit, whilst an average glass of wine will cost you 2-3 units. A lemonade or soft drink with a shot of vodka or similar strength spirits will set you back another unit.

The more units your body needs to process the worse your sleep will be. Try to ensure that you're not over 1-2 units or 1-2 hours of alcohol digestion when you go to sleep (although it would be best to cut the alcohol entirely). Please bear in mind these are rough approximations – a faster metabolism can deal with alcohol quickly and visa-verse.

Chapter 3: Sleep Hygiene

Sleep hygiene isn't about body odor – it's all the small ways you can ensure your sleeping routine is as healthy as possible. We have already talked about avoiding bright lights in the evening, but often people fail to consider all the smaller, forgettable small sources of light.

For example, LED's from electrical devices which are on standby can add a huge amount of artificial light into a room. Likewise, your curtains should block out nearly *all* the light from the windows. This means that they need to properly cover up all your window space in addition to being thick and heavy enough to block out *all* light.

On the same vein, your need to find that Goldilocks temperature where you are comfortable – neither too hot nor too cold. If you find yourself frequently too warm, try lighter sheets and duvets, opening the window or implementing some type of ventilation and air flow. If you are too cold, wear pajamas, close the window, use a hot water bottle and so on.

The sound is another sleep hygiene issue. Obviously, there is only so much you can do about inconsiderate neighbors or background city noise, but ear plugs can compensate for poor manners. Otherwise, consider ambient noise from electrical devices or the ticking of clocks and all the small, but perhaps partially unnoticed sounds, that may prevent you from relaxing entirely.

Chapter 4: Associate Your Bed With Sleep

The mind is a subtle device. Psychologists have discovered the more you use your bed and bedroom for other activities apart from sleep and sexual activity, the harder it becomes to fall asleep when you actually need to.

Non-consciously you associate particular places and items, with certain actions and states of mind. Whenever you watch TV in bed, or read, or even just lay awake thinking to yourself, you are giving your brain mixed messages. Instead, if you only sleep in your bedroom, your brain makes the link between sleeping and your bedroom. This means that when you next go to sleep, you start to relax and enter sleep faster and more peacefully.

A similar argument explains why trying to force yourself to go to sleep by laying in your bed doesn't work. If you become frustrated and stressed about *trying* to get to sleep, then you will start making a mental link between your frustration and your bed. This is obviously a bad thing.

Therefore, if you find yourself simply unable to go to sleep, then leave your bed and bedroom and go do something else. Of course, hopping onto a computer or watching TV (especially in your bedroom) isn't the solution. Instead, do some light reading, listen to peaceful music or any other activity that isn't mentally or physically taxing in a different room. Eventually, your frustrations will start to subside and you will naturally become tired again. Now go back to your bed.

As a related note, avoid clocks and anything that tells you the time. Seeing the minutes pass by painfully slowly and gaining an awareness of just how much sleep you might be missing is a fantastic way to stress yourself out.

If you leave a phone or clock by your bedside, you'll have the temptation to look at it anytime you wake up, which will start to make you feel more awake. If you need a phone or clock in your room, put it on a surface that isn't in reach from your bed, and ensure the clock isn't facing your direction. This also has the added benefit of forcing you to get out of bed to answer the annoyance of your alarm in the morning, which helps you avoid snoozing.

In some weird Zen-cryptic way, the only way to get to sleep is not to try. Trying to go to sleep, prevents the process entirely. Rather, you should divert all your efforts to making yourself relax and you'll drift off naturally (relaxation techniques will be covered later).

Leaving your bed when you're not sleeping also goes for snoozing and trying to go back to sleep in the morning. If you find yourself awake and you cannot fall back asleep immediately, you need to leave your bed.

Generally speaking, when you drift in and out of sleep, you tend to only go into a very light sleep and fail to rejuvenate. Therefore, even if you still feel a little sleep or tired, you probably won't get much by lounging in your bed in some half-conscious, half-asleep state.

Rather, by getting out of bed the moment you wake, you ensure you keep the bed a sacred place for sleeping, sex and nothing else. It also ensures that you are tired when it comes around to the evening that day, which should help you sleep like a log during the next night.

Chapter 5: Challenge Negative Thoughts

Insomnia has strong connections to depression, anxiety and stress. These are complex problems of their own accord and if you think you are suffering from any of mental health problems, seek professional help. Nonetheless, positive thinking, whilst not a solitary solution, is a great start to improving your emotional health, which in turn can help alleviate insomnia.

In particular, it's important to tackle negative thoughts and negative thought patterns, rationally and logically. People who struggle with insomnia often fail to approach their dilemma from a calm, structured approach. Insomniacs often lose hope entirely and become despondent owing to ingrained negative thinking habits.

For example, one negative thinking habit is the tendency to develop negative expectations. In regards to insomnia, going to bed with the expectation that you are going to have an awkward and difficult night's sleep is going to prevent you from relaxing and make you feel stressed. Even though you might have had chronic trouble going to sleep in the past, you need to approach each evening with a fresh mindset.

If you find yourself starting to dwell on a negative expectation, you either need to distract your thoughts on another matter, or you need to challenge the thought. For example, if the thought *"I'll never get a good nights sleep again"* occurs (or a similar thought) you need to say to yourself *'never say never'* or *'perhaps today will be different'*.

Other common negative thought patterns include the tendency to exaggerate. Mentally exclaiming that you'll never get a good sleep again is *obviously* hyperbole. You know it is probably not true, but making exaggerated statements have a big impact on our state of mind. You need to keep your thoughts grounded. Perhaps you will have a bad night's sleep, perhaps not. Either way, there's no need to make over-top statements of despair – they serve no purpose and they help no-one.

Additionally, avoid fortune telling, hopelessness and catastrophizing. Fortune telling can be summarized as believing you *know* a negative outcome will occur (*"I'm not getting a good night's sleep tonight"*), whilst hopelessness is the pattern of believing there is no solution or alternative (*"There's nothing I can do..."*). Catastrophizing is the tendency to believe negative outcomes are more important than they actually are (*'Everything is ruined'.*)

You need to prevent or challenge yourself whenever you are thinking this way about your insomnia and your lack of sleep. In fact, challenging or distracting yourself from these thought patterns is a good practice for every aspect of your life.

Chapter 6: Breathing Relaxation

As previously mentioned the key to going to sleep peacefully is being relaxed. Yet most of us are never relaxed and even attempting to relax can be stressful. Owing to this learning how to manually calm yourself through breathing techniques can be a fantastic way to make sure you fall asleep quickly.

There are many types of breathing techniques, although the one most commonly used for relaxation is deep breathing. Depending on your state of mind, you actually breathe differently. During exercise and whenever you feel anxious or stressed, your breath becomes shallow, tight and centers in the chest.

However, when you are fully relaxed your breath should originate from the diaphragm and lower stomach. As you might expect, more people are closer to the shallow type of breathing than the deep type of breathing. Yet if you take a few moments every now and then to force yourself to breathe deeply, deep breathing can become a habit and you will find yourself feeling calmer & grounded.

To start a deep breathing session, lie down on your bed and place your lower hand on your stomach. You can sit upright if you wish, however, ensure that you are sitting in a comfortable position (it is rather hard to relax if your back or legs are in pain).

Expunge all the air from your lungs. By emptying your lungs of all air first, you make it easier to breathe to your maximum capacity. Breathe in *slowly*. Your inhalation should take 2-3 seconds to fully draw in all the available air – this might feel slightly uncomfortable at first, but after a few dozen breaths, it should start to feel more natural. When you inhale, you should feel your lower belly expand. If this doesn't happen naturally, force the movement to give your diaphragm room to expand. After your inhalation, pause for just a second.

The temptation to automatically release the breath will be high, but resist. Holding the breath in your lungs allows more oxygen to enter your bloodstream and release more carbon dioxide. It also gives you time to feel the natural desire to exhale to grow, which should make the following exhalation fluid.

Exhale, also taking between 2-3 seconds to allow yourself to fully release all the air in your lungs. When all the air has been released, pause for 1 second before you next inhalation. You should feel your diaphragm deflate. If it doesn't force the movement once more, pulling your stomach inwards. After a lifetime of poor breathing habits, the deep inhalation, and exhalation of the breath is difficult and you might need to push and pull the muscles to act in the way you want.

Keep breathing in this deep manner for at least several minutes. You can keep breathing for as long as you like. In fact, if you are lying down when you start, you might find yourself drifting off into wonderland once you have started to relax.

Chapter 7: Exercise

People who exercise tend to fall asleep faster, have more restorative sleep and tend not to awake earlier in the morning. The exercise doesn't even have to be particularly intense, with even 30 minute walks demonstrating a significant effect. However, the exercise does need to be aerobic, with activities such as weight lifting or sprinting not impacting sleep routines significantly.

In fact, moderate intensity exercise seems to be better than high-intensity exercise, with long distance running actually having less impact than a milder jog or small walk. Likewise, you probably want to avoid exercise for at least for 3-4 hours before you actually go to sleep.

So why does exercise seem to affect insomnia? The exact causal mechanism isn't known. One theory suggests that the increase in body temperature and subsequent decrease in temperature post-workout promotes falling asleep. Alternatively, it is known that exercise tackles many of the causes of insomnia – anxiety, stress, and depression – which will obviously have an impact. Finally, it may also change the timing of your circadian rhythm or 'body clock' adjusting it back to a more convenient timing so you feel tired when you should.

Exercise isn't a quick fix for your insomnia problems, however – you'll need to consistently exercise for at least three, thirty-minute sessions per week for several weeks to see a large improvement. Furthermore, you are probably going to see less benefit if you already exercise frequently, with the largest improvements seen in the sedentary and elderly.

Chapter 8: Daily Closure

One reason why people struggle to go to sleep is because they are unsatisfied with their day. This might be because they failed to achieve goals they set for themselves or because there is some problem or issue that has been left unresolved. Alternatively, there are often emotional blocks which prevent us from being fully content.

You can overcome this dissatisfaction by taking some steps every evening to provide closure for your day. For example, one recommended activity is to write a to-do list for the next day before you go to sleep. This ensures that any nagging worries or responsibilities are addressed before you go to sleep, rather than pop up in your mind as you are trying to relax.

Moreover, it can be useful to mentally re-enact your day, visualizing all your actions and experiences from when you woke up to your current point in time. This isn't an opportunity to criticize yourself or feel inadequate about any of the decisions you have made. Rather this should be a time where you concentrate on all the sensations and feelings of your day – the taste of your breakfast and the glass of orange juice you washed it down with. Your walk to work (and so on).

You should also make an effort to try and remember all the little details. How many slices of toast did you have? What time did you set off in the morning? How was the weather? By focusing on all these details, you distract your mind from thoughts that may be keeping you awake whilst also giving your mind ample material and stimulation to start dreaming.

Chapter 9: Full Body Relaxation

There are many more techniques than just deep breathing you can use to relax. Full body relaxation is the phrase for several mental visualizations and practices aimed at completely and utterly relaxing the body. Typically if your mind and body are stressed than your flight or fight response is activated and a flood of hormones and chemicals which prepare your body for action. This is fantastic if you want to fight a lion with a spear, but it is awful if you want to get some shut-eye.

The most common full body relaxation technique is progressive muscle relaxation. In this technique, you focus your awareness in each part of the body, in turn, tensing it and relaxing the muscles progressively. This is useful as by focusing on the body you distract yourself from all the ruminating and brooding that may be occurring in your mind. Alternatively, tensing the muscles helps the muscles themselves to relax once released, which is useful if you are feeling stressed and overwhelmed.

Start by focusing on all your attention on your toes on your right foot. Tense all the muscles in your toe and hold this tension for 10-15 seconds before releasing. Move up to your ankle, calves, buttocks, back, shoulders, biceps, triceps, neck and facial muscles, tensing and releasing all these muscle groups in turn. Next repeat the process for all the muscles groups on the left-hand side of the body, working all the way down to your right foot.

End the process by tensing all the muscles in your body for 10-15 seconds before releasing.

If you struggle to tense the left and the right side of the body separately, then you can tense both sides of the body simultaneously. The more you practice this technique, the more subtle and refined your concentration will become. Gradually it should become easier to hold your focus on one particular area of the body without distraction, and you should eventually be able to focus on smaller muscles groups at a time.

The entire routine should take no longer than 5-10 minutes to fulfill. However, you can find yourself in a deeper state of relaxation if you complete the full body muscle relaxation 2-3 times before you allow your mind to wander.

It is best if you complete the muscle relaxation at the same time every day – this will condition your mind to relax at that given point. Many people choose to do a full body relaxation before they go to sleep.

Another similar technique is a full body scan. With a full body scan, you simply focus on all the areas of your body in turn without tensing the muscles – you just observe   what sensations come to mind whilst your attention dwells on that area.

With full body relaxation, you might also want to focus on your breath as you focus on your body as well. If any part of your body is experiencing pain, don't shy away your attention from that area. Lean into the pain and just gradually explore how it feels. This may be uncomfortable, but if you learn to stop resisting the sensation then you will eventually be able to relax, even if you are in pain. Whilst in an ideal world everyone would be pain-free, learning to cope with pain is often the best realistic compromise.

Chapter 10: Visualization

Visualization is another effective relaxation technique that can be used to combat insomnia. By imagining a peaceful environment, you both distract your mind from worries and doubts that are keeping you awake and you relax the mind with gentle imagery.

The key to visualization is to make your imagination vivid and detailed. Start by thinking of a place or environment that you find peaceful. This could be from a memory or place you know, but if nothing comes to mind, you can construct your own environment.

Popular choices include a lakeside cabin, a beach hut, an isolated mountain retreat, a tidy and clean room or a field underneath a starlit sky. However, your places don't have to be scenic or natural – if a football stadium or a bustling high street is where you find yourself most at ease, just roll with it.

Now that you have an idea, you need to embellish the concept with the power of all your senses. What do you hear? What do you feel against your skin? Is it daytime or nighttime? What can you see in the distance? What do you taste? Consider all the different feelings and sensations that would arise if you were really there.

Once you have fully decorated the world your are imagining, take a minute just to observe and let everything sink in.

Sometimes this visualization is enough to send you to sleep, but more often than not you will need to make a journey in your visualized world. This journey helps really focus your brain – if you just imagine a static scene, your mind will have a temptation to just wander back to all those thoughts keeping you awake. By doing something, you make the visualization even stronger.

Your journey or activity can be whatever you want, although it should be consistent with your world. If you imagine yourself in a beach hut, for example, you might visualize yourself walking across the sand and feeling the waves rush against your feet. If you are walking down a busy high street, you could imagine yourself window shopping or find somewhere to buy a drink and just observe people walking by.

Sometimes people find it helpful to imagine some symbolic representation of tiredness or sleep within their visualization, that they embrace. For example, if you are on the beach you can imagine walking into the ocean, with you feeling a little more sleepy and relaxed as you go deeper until you are completely submerged.

Or if you are sitting on a mountain, you can imagine watching the sunset, with you slowly drifting off to sleep as the sun sinks into the horizon. It doesn't really matter what you visualize as long you visualize it deeply.

Conclusion

By having finished this guide, you have learned ten ways to alleviate your insomnia. The first chapter informed you about the importance of having a sleep schedule, which adjusts your biological systems that manage your sleep. Meanwhile, the second chapter reminded you to be wary of caffeine, nicotine, and alcohol. Many people are vaguely aware of the negative impacts these substances can have on their sleep but underestimate the sheer extent of havoc they can unleash.

Moreover, the third chapter made you aware of the various ways you can improve your sleep hygiene and the fourth chapter emphasized the importance of conditioning your mind to associate your bed with sleep. In chapter 5 you learned to tackle negative thinking habits whilst chapter 6 taught you how to calm your body and mind via the breath.

Chapter 7 re-affirmed the value of a good pulse-raising bout of exercise, whilst chapter 8 gave you a couple of ways to provide some much-needed closure to your days. Chapter 9 inducted you into the usage of full body relaxation techniques, whilst chapter 10 gave you the scenic route with visualization methods.

Yet, if there is one message you should take home from this guide, it isn't a specific technique or snippet of advice. It is that insomnia is a solvable problem. You shouldn't accept those endless, restless nights or the array of difficulties they can cause you.

Curing your insomnia may not happen overnight and it does take effort, yet if you apply the techniques in this guide, you should find yourself consistency improving the quantity and quality of your sleep.

www.ingramcontent.com/pod-product-compliance
Lightning Source LLC
Chambersburg PA
CBHW071321280526
45788CB00004B/1974